Christophe MALOMALO LIMANGA

Mortality during tuberculosis treatment in the DRC

Christophe MALOMALO LIMANGA

Mortality during tuberculosis treatment in the DRC

What factors influence mortality during the intensive phase of anti-tuberculosis treatment?

ScienciaScripts

Imprint
Any brand names and product names mentioned in this book are subject to trademark, brand or patent protection and are trademarks or registered trademarks of their respective holders. The use of brand names, product names, common names, trade names, product descriptions etc. even without a particular marking in this work is in no way to be construed to mean that such names may be regarded as unrestricted in respect of trademark and brand protection legislation and could thus be used by anyone.

Cover image: www.ingimage.com

This book is a translation from the original published under ISBN 978-620-8-82397-9.

Publisher:
Sciencia Scripts
is a trademark of
Dodo Books Indian Ocean Ltd. and OmniScriptum S.R.L publishing group

120 High Road, East Finchley, London, N2 9ED, United Kingdom
Str. Armeneasca 28/1, office 1, Chisinau MD-2012, Republic of Moldova, Europe
Managing Directors: Ieva Konstantinova, Victoria Ursu
info@omniscriptum.com

Printed at: see last page
ISBN: 978-620-8-98980-4

DEDICATION

To my very dear Parents : MALOMALO BONAMA Jean and BALEMA BONGALE KOWANA Marie

To my brothers and sisters MALOMALO ONOYENA Joël, MALOMALO SILIKA John, MALOMALO BAIYA Sarah and MALOMALO BAITA Boni.

To my future wife

To all those who love the Lord Jesus

Christophe MALOMALO LIMANGA

ACKNOWLEDGEMENTS

There is a tradition in higher and university education whereby at the end of the first or second cycle a scientific paper is presented by the student to sanction or crown his or her academic career.

As an exception to the rule, we have carried out research with the help of a number of people whose names we will not reveal.

So, first of all, we would like to express our gratitude to the Lord, Jesus Christ, the Almighty God, master of time and circumstance, for the goodness and mercy he has freely offered us and for keeping us in good health until the end of this work.

Our most sincere thanks go in general to all the academic authorities at the University of Kisangani (UNIKIS) and to all the lecturers at the Faculty of Medicine and Pharmacy, because this work is the fruit of the teaching we received from them and which made us what we are.

We would also like to thank in particular Professor Dr J. Paulin MBO MUKONKOLE, the director of this work, for his availability, his patience, his comments and observations of great scientific importance for the successful progress of my research, which has been of great importance to me. I would like to express my very sincere thanks to him.

Our most sincere thanks go to the supervisor, Dr KAZADI MUSAKAYI Daniel, who in spite of his multiple occupations, agreed to supervise the present work and was always there to advise us and guide us towards the right path.

Our deepest gratitude goes to our Reverend Pastor KABAMBA Christophore for the good guidance of our souls in the Lord and to the honourable deacons, Emmanuel BAMBU, Alou MUNGAMBA, LIKUNDE Joseph...

Our special thanks go to our parents Jean MALOMALO BONAMA and Marie BALEMA BONGALE KOWANA, for their sacrifices and invaluable support which led to the completion of this work.

We would like to thank our brothers and sisters Joël MALOMALO, John MALOMALO, Sarah KASHAMA MALOMALO and Boni MALMALO, Félix PONYO, Patrick ISAMENE, Keren BONGALE, Pauliane LITWASE and Rebecca KOPI for all their support.

To our aunts and uncles, SILIKA LITOFE OSHISHEMO Joël, Mardoché BALEMA, Angel YAKANGA and to our grandmother Pauliane LITWASE LILALA, we say thank you for your support.

We would like to express our gratitude to the couple Jacques Riverain LOFEMBA for their support.

To our wrestling colleagues: Nathan MAGO, Freddy MOMBULA, Laureine BAYILONGO, Astrid KISUBI, Grâce KAMABU, Dorcas NASIBU, Samuel KITENGE, LOLLIS John, Jean Claude MULUMBILA, Héritier WALISI and others. Thank you for your advice and encouragement.

A to you, our brothers and sisters in Christ: Dr LOFOLI BOKOTA, Patrick KAOMBE, Anne WABI AMUDA, Merlin WABI, Dieu-Merci BATIUNDE, Franck BOINA, Esperance ZEDE, La Rose MONDEMA, Myriam BAZI etc. we say thank you.

We would like to express our gratitude to all those who have helped us in one way or another.

Christophe MALOMALO LIMANGA

SUMMARY

INTRODUCTION

Tuberculosis is a contagious disease that is a major cause of ill health and one of the leading causes of death worldwide. The aim of this study was to determine the case-fatality rate associated with tuberculosis and to identify the factors associated with this case-fatality.

METHODOLOGY

We conducted a longitudinal study of a cohort of adults infected with tuberculosis and undergoing anti-tuberculosis treatment. Our sample consisted of 171 patients undergoing anti-TB treatment in the CDTs we selected during our study period from 15 June 2022 to 15 April 2023.

RESULTS

Mortality in the intensive phase of tuberculosis treatment was high (11.11%).

Age > 55 years (RR = 3.39; CI = 1.57 - 13.36), time to consultation > 30 days, smoking (RR = 2.38; CI = 1.51 -13.75), alcoholism (RR = 2.22 ; CI = 1.50 - 12.99), dyspnoea (RR = 1.92; CI = 1.84 - 6.41), pallor (RR = 2.41; CI = 1.51 - 8.35), dizziness (RR = 2.32; CI = 1.42 - 14.12), bedridden (RR = 1.7 ; CI = 1.43 - 13.15), profound deterioration in general condition (RR = 3.01; CI = 1.42 - 6.38), positive HIV serology (RR = 3.62; CI = 1.21 - 11.85), and BMI < 18.5 (RR = 2.08; CI = 1.46 - 1.55) were the best predictors of mortality or risk factors for mortality in the intensive phase of tuberculosis treatment. On the other hand, delay of consultation ≤ 30 days was a protective factor (RR = 0.43; CI = 0.22 - 0.88).

CONCLUSION

Mortality during the intensive phase of treatment was high. Patients aged over 55, those with a delay in consultation of more than 30 days, patients with a history of smoking or alcoholism, people living with HIV, patients presenting with dyspnoea, pallor, vertigo, bed rest, profound deterioration in general condition and patients with a BMI of less than 18.5 kg/m^2should be monitored with particular care, or even referred to a centre of excellence to reduce the number of deaths.

KEYWORDS: *Tuberculosis, Risk factor, Intensive phase, Mortality*

INTRODUCTION

1. Issues

Tuberculosis is a communicable disease that is one of the major causes of ill health and a leading cause of death worldwide. (1) Until the emergence of the COVID-19 pandemic, tuberculosis was the leading cause of death attributable to a single infectious agent, ahead of HIV/AIDS. (1)

Tuberculosis is caused by the bacillus *Mycobacterium tuberculosis*, which is spread mainly through the air when people with tuberculosis cough the bacteria into the air. The disease generally affects the lungs (pulmonary tuberculosis), but can also affect other organs. Almost a quarter of the world's population is infected with *M. tuberculosis*. (1) (2)

Globally, an estimated 10 million people (CI: 8.9-11.0 million) contracted TB in 2019, a number that has been declining very slowly in recent years. TB deaths in 2019 were estimated at 1.2 million (CI: 1.1-1.3 million) among HIV-negative people (down from 1.7 million in 2000), with an additional 208,000 deaths (CI: 177,000 -242,000) among HIV-positive people (down from 678,000 in 2000). Males (aged ≥15 years) accounted for 56% of all people developing TB in 2019; females and children (aged <15 years) accounted for 32% and 12% of cases respectively. Of all TB cases, 8.2% were people living with HIV. (2)

In 2020, with COVID-19, years of progress in reducing the number of TB deaths worldwide were reversed. The number of deaths worldwide among people seronegative for HIV rose from 1.2 million in 2019 to 1.3 million and the number of HIV-TB co-infected deaths rose from 208,000 in 2019 to 214,000 in 2020. (1)

According to the World Health Organisation's (WHO) report on the leading causes of death in the world in 2020, tuberculosis was the 13th leading cause of death in the world and the leading cause of death due to a single infectious agent. (1)

Geographically, in 2020, the world's tuberculosis cases were distributed as follows: most tuberculosis cases were recorded in the WHO Regions of South-East Asia (43%), Africa (25%) and the Western Pacific (18%), with smaller percentages in the WHO Regions of the Eastern Mediterranean (8.3%), the Americas (3.0%) and Europe (2.3%). The 30 countries with a high burden of tuberculosis accounted for 86% of the total estimated incident cases worldwide, and eight of these countries accounted for two-thirds of the world total: India (26%), China (8.5%), Indonesia (8.4%), the Philippines (6.0%), Pakistan (5.8%), Nigeria (4.6%), Bangladesh (3.6%) and South Africa (3.3%). (1)

According to WHO estimates, 270,000 people fell ill with TB in the DRC in 2018, equivalent to an incidence of 321 cases per 100,000 people. Of these, 31,000 were people living with HIV (PLHIV), or 11.5%. Of the 270,000 people thought to have fallen ill with TB, only 171,682 were diagnosed in 2018, meaning that 100,000 (37%) of those affected remained undiagnosed and untreated. The WHO also estimates that around 53,000 people died from the disease, i.e. 63 deaths per 100,000 people. (3) In 2020, the incidence of tuberculosis in the DRC was 319 cases per 100,000 inhabitants. (4) In 2021, the DRC's National Tuberculosis Control Programme (PNLT) reported a total of 216,690 cases of TB in all its forms. (5)

Several studies carried out on tuberculosis in Africa and around the world have shown that most deaths occur in the first two months of treatment, i.e. the intensive phase. (6; 7; 8; 9; 10; 11; 12; 13; 14; 15)

Around the world, a number of studies have looked at the results of tuberculosis treatment by examining the factors associated with mortality in patients with tuberculosis. These studies have shown that these risk factors vary greatly depending on the environment.

With regard to industrialised countries, N. Lefebvre et al, in their study in Europe, demonstrated that delayed diagnosis and treatment are risk factors for mortality in tuberculosis. (16) According to the study conducted by I.S. Pradipta et al in the Netherlands in 2018, the predictive factors for mortality were age greater than or equal to 74 years, combined pulmonary and extra-pulmonary tuberculosis, tuberculosis of the central nervous system, miliary tuberculosis, drug addiction and renal failure/dialysis. (17)

With regard to developing countries, Gelaw et al, in a study carried out in Ethiopia in 2021, found that anaemia is a risk factor for death from tuberculosis. (18) In the study conducted in Rabat, Morocco, by Hicham J. et al, the terrain, delayed diagnosis and treatment side-effects were the main risk factors for mortality in patients hospitalised for pulmonary tuberculosis. (19) Adil Sbayi, et al, in a study conducted in Morocco in 2020, demonstrated that in cases of extrapulmonary tuberculosis, age is significantly associated with tuberculosis-related mortality. (20) In Kenya, the study conducted by Osman A. Abdullahi et al in 2019 found that age, female sex, extrapulmonary TB, malnutrition, HIV infection and year of diagnosis were significantly associated with mortality. (6) Muhammad Osman et al demonstrated in their study conducted in South Africa in 2021 that age greater than or equal to 65 years, positive HIV serology, a history of tuberculosis treatment and extrapulmonary tuberculosis presented an increased risk of death. (21) In the DRC, Henegar C et al, in 2012, found that high mortality during the first months of treatment was linked to delayed diagnosis, extrapulmonary TB and bacilloscopy-negative TB, as well as HIV-TB co-infection. (22) In the city of Kisangani, the work carried out by LILOLO in 2018 found that age over 45, a bedridden attitude and a long duration of illness before the start of treatment were factors linked to mortality. (23)

In view of the above, we proposed to carry out this study in order to answer the following question:

What is the case fatality rate for tuberculosis and what factors are associated with it?

2. Objectives

2.1. General objective

- Helping to reduce tuberculosis-related mortality in Kisangani.

2.2. Specific objectives

- To determine the mortality rate linked to tuberculosis in the city of Kisangani in the post-CVID period.
- To determine the risk factors for tuberculosis mortality in the city of Kisangani and the link between these factors and mortality.

3. Assumptions

Given that we are in a developing country, and given the factors found by others who have worked before us, we have adopted the following hypotheses:

a) Mortality in the intensive phase of tuberculosis treatment is high in Kisangani ;

b) Age $\geq$ 55 years, HIV-positive status, smoking, alcoholism, diabetes, cardiovascular disease, dyspnoea, haemoptysis, bedridden attitude on admission, delay in diagnosis and BMI < 18.5 were risk factors for mortality in the intensive phase of tuberculosis treatment.

4. Interest in the work

By determining the factors linked to mortality from tuberculosis in Kisangani, this work is of interest because it can help TDC nurses to identify patients at risk of death at the time of diagnosis, and to refer these patients in good time for proper management.

5. Labour division

Apart from the introduction and conclusion, our work comprises four chapters:

- Chapter 1: General information on tuberculosis
- Chapter two: Materials and methods
- Chapter three: Presentation of results
- Chapter four: Discussion

Chapter 1: General information on tuberculosis

1.1. Definition and aetiology

1.1.1. Definition

Tuberculosis (TB) is an infectious disease caused by *Mycobacterium tuberculosis* (MTB) or Koch's bacillus (B.K). The contagiousness of a case of tuberculosis is determined by the concentration of bacilli inside the lungs and their spread in the surrounding air. Patients with microscopy-positive pulmonary tuberculosis are the most contagious cases. (24)

1.1.2. Etiopathogenesis

1.1.2.1. Agent :

Tuberculosis is a bacterial infectious disease. The main bacterium responsible for the disease is ***Mycobacterium tuberculosis*** or Koch's bacillus (BK), isolated by Robert Koch in 1882. It is responsible for almost all human tuberculosis.

On direct examination of the smear, it appears as an acid-alcohol-resistant bacillus (Ziehl stain) or fluorescent (auramine stain). M. tuberculosis has the property of surviving only in humans or animals. It is therefore an obligate pathogen.

Two other varieties exist: Mycobacterium bovis can exceptionally be transmitted to humans through unpasteurised milk from a sick cow; and Mycobacterium africanum is another variety that sometimes exists in West African countries. These three species are "tuberculous mycobacteria" and make up the "***tuberculosis complex***".

There are non-tuberculous mycobacteria, or atypical mycobacteria, which are often non-pathogenic due to their low virulence. However, they can give rise to clinical manifestations (pulmonary, lymph nodes, skin or bone) that mimic those of tuberculosis. These are known as ***mycobacteriosis***. These opportunistic mycobacteria cause disease, particularly in countries with a low prevalence of tuberculosis and in immunocompromised patients. (25)

1.1.2.2. Source and method of contamination *(25)*

1.1.2.2.1. Source of contamination :

The main source of contamination is humans suffering from bacilliferous pulmonary tuberculosis.

In exceptional cases, cattle or sheep with tuberculous mastitis (M. bovis) may also be affected.

1.1.2.2.2. Mode of contamination :

The main route of contamination is airborne: when coughing, talking, laughing, sneezing or singing, a person with pulmonary tuberculosis emits fine droplets of secretions known as "Flügge droplets". As these droplets evaporate, they give rise to a microaerosol containing only a few mycobacteria (droplet nuclei).

1.1.2.3. Reactions following primary contamination *(25)*

The characteristics of the tubercle bacillus determine the development of tuberculosis infection and disease.

1. It is an obligate aerobic bacillus, whose development depends on the availability of oxygen.
2. It multiplies slowly (once every 24 hours).
3. It multiplies in both extracellular and intracellular environments.

The primo-contaminated human organism resists bacillary attack poorly for the first 6 weeks.

When airborne germs reach the alveoli, they multiply there, even within the macrophages, and cause the development of a local pneumonic reaction, ***the primary chancre***, generally located in the basal and anterior zones.

The germs and macrophages are carried along the lymphatic tracts and cause ***satellite adenopathies*** to form in the homolateral hilum, from where they travel to the thoracic duct and the blood, causing haematogenous dissemination. Cellular immunity develops after 4 to 6 weeks. Following phagocytosis of the bacilli by macrophages, bacillus antigens are released. The antigens trigger the activation of non-specific lymphocytes, which become specific CD4 and CD8 lymphocytes. These specific lymphocytes support immunity in tuberculosis. These T lymphocytes, sensitised by M. tuberculosis antigens, activate macrophages, which become capable of killing many tubercle bacilli. The bacilli disappear and the lesions they have caused are largely reabsorbed.

However, some bacilli respond to this aggression by reducing their metabolism and going into a dormant state, which allows them to survive in the lesions for years and, once a normal metabolism has been re-established, to become the starting point for "*endogenous reactivations*", especially in well-oxygenated areas and those where there is a local immune deficiency.

After the onset of cellular immunity, subsequent exogenous reinfections are often abortive.

At the same time as specific cellular immunity develops, a delayed cellular hypersensitivity to tuberculin proteins develops under the action of other M. tuberculosis antigens.

Sensitised T lymphocytes multiply and secrete lymphokines. These sensitise the skin to tuberculo-proteins (tuberculin reactions). But they also have a toxic action on the tissues, causing inflammatory reactions and tuberculosis necrosis or caseation.

When the hypersensitivity reaction occurs earlier or is more intense than cellular immunity, tuberculosis infection is followed by tuberculosis disease (patent primary infection).

Immunity secondary to the formation of circulating antibodies plays a marginal role in tuberculosis, because mycobacteria are resistant to the direct effect of antibodies and complement. However, the existence of these antibodies is the basis of research into new serological diagnostic techniques for tuberculosis.

1.1.2.4. Development of tuberculosis after infection *(24)*

The risk of developing the disease is highest in the period immediately following infection, but persists throughout life. Of those infected, 10% may develop active TB disease, while around 90% will never develop active TB disease, unless their immunity is seriously compromised.

Tuberculosis develops in the human body in two stages: Tuberculosis infection: this occurs when a person is exposed to the bacilli of a contagious tuberculosis patient. This infection is usually asymptomatic, except in the case of primary infection or primary tuberculosis in children. The course of the disease depends on the immune system, i.e. the body's defences. Tuberculosis disease: this is when the symptoms of tuberculosis disease appear in the infected person.

1.1.2.5. The impact of HIV on tuberculosis and tuberculosis on HIV infection *(24)*

HIV infection leads to widespread destruction of the body's defence mechanisms.

HIV infection has an amplifying effect on tuberculosis. This is because it :

- Promotes the development of progressive TB in recent infections (primary TB);
- Accelerates the development of latent infections into progressive TB;
- Promotes the reactivation of an old latent TB infection;
- Favours recurrence of TB (endogenous reactivation or exogenous reinfection);

- Increases the risk of TB transmission (increase in the infectious pool);
- Increases pauci bacillary pulmonary forms and extra pulmonary forms.

Tuberculosis is the leading cause of death among people living with HIV. This can be explained by the fact that :

- Accelerates the progression of HIV infection to AIDS;
- Significantly reduces the life expectancy of HIV-positive subjects

1.1.2.6. Resistance to anti-tuberculosis drugs *(24)*

The existence of a number of drug-resistant bacilli within a susceptible bacillary strain is a natural phenomenon. In the case of tuberculosis, the selection of resistant mutants secondary to the prescription of inappropriate therapeutic regimens, or following poor compliance with treatment by patients, leads to the multiplication of these mutants and the appearance of strains with acquired resistance to one or more antibiotics.

1.1.2.7. Tuberculosis in children *(24)*

Diagnosing tuberculosis in children is not easy, and most providers do not look for it due to a lack of guidelines and resources in the field.

According to the WHO, tuberculosis in children accounts for 10-20% of all tuberculosis cases in high-prevalence countries such as the DRC.

1.2. Diagnosis of tuberculosis (24)

1.2.1. Clinical signs of pulmonary tuberculosis

The clinical signs suggestive of tuberculosis are :

Table II Clinical signs of tuberculosis

Cough	Weight loss	Dyspnoea
Fever (temperature)	Anorexia	Chest pain
Night sweats	Asthenia	Haemoptysis

The most common clinical signs of tuberculosis (cough, dyspnoea and sputum) are not very specific and may suggest a large number of conditions (see chapter on the respiratory health approach). However, in countries with a high prevalence of tuberculosis, such as the DRC, the diagnosis of tuberculosis should always be made in the presence of these clinical signs.

1.2.2. Diagnosis of extra pulmonary tuberculosis (EPT)

Whatever the suspected site, samples will be collected for smears and/or culture to diagnose the PET scan.

Clinical approach to the diagnosis of extra pulmonary tuberculosis.

TableII Clinical approach to the diagnosis of extra pulmonary tuberculosis.

Anatomical sites	Clinical presentation	Diagnostic approach
TB in lymph nodes	• Enlargement of a lymph node ; • Asymmetrical and painless; • Most often in the cervical region	• Fine needle aspiration if possible for GeneXpert, culture and histology; • IDR generally positive ; • If the axillary lymph node is on the same side as the BCG, think of BCGitis after vaccination.
Pleural TB (older children and adolescents)	• Cough; • Softness on percussion and reduction of respiratory noise; • Chest pain ; • X-ray: diffuse, homogeneous opacity in one hemi thorax.	• Chest X-ray ; • Pleural puncture (WBC, protein, culture...) : • Treat for TB if the puncture fluid is high in protein and lymphocytes are predominant; • If purulent fluid, consider the possibility of empyema; • Thoracic and/or ericardial ultrasound

Anatomical sites	Clinical presentation	Diagnostic approach
Meningeal TB	• Headaches, irritability/ behavioural problems ; • Vomiting, lethargy/altered consciousness, even coma; • Convulsions, stiff neck, bulging fontanel (infants), cranial nerve paralysis with strabismus.	Lumbar puncture with cytology, biochemistry and culture of the CSF: A high cytology with lymphocytic predominance (may be neutrophilic at the beginning); with high protein and chlorine levels are in favour of TB.
Abdominal TB	• Abdominal bloating: ascites or abdominal masses; • Shortness of breath ; • The most common site is the ileo-caecal region. It may present as a palpable mass in the right lower quadrant and/or with signs of intestinal obstruction, perforation or malabsorption.	• Abdominal puncture with cytology, biochemistry and culture of the puncture fluid: TB if high cytology with lymphocytic predominance and high protein content; • Abdominal ultrasound ; • CT Scan

Anatomical sites	Clinical presentation	Diagnostic approach
Spinal TB (Pott's disease) and osteoarticular TB	• Typically occurs within 6 to 36 months of primary infection; • The most common site is the spine, followed by the knee knee, hip and ankle joints; • The following signs indicate TB in the bones or joints joints: - sudden onset of angulation of the spine ; - progressive weakness of the lower limbs - joint effusions; - Progression of the disease may lead to destruction of the joint, with or without abscess.	X-ray of the suspected area ; - Ultrasound ; - Biopsy ; - Joint puncture: with cytology, biochemistry and culture of the puncture fluid: TB if high cytology with predominance of lymphocytes and high protein content;
Pericardial TB	• Heart failure ; • Muffling of heart sounds ; • Shortness of breath ; • Cough, chest pain ; • Dizziness ; • Fainting ; • Acceleration of the heart rate	• Chest X-ray ; • Cardiac ultrasound ; • Pericardial puncture with cytology, biochemistry and culture of the puncture fluid: TB if elevated cells with lymphocytic predominance and high protein content.

1.2.3. Technique for diagnosing tuberculosis (24)

1.2.3.1. Microscopy for BAARs

We have two main methods:

- The Ziehl-Neelsen hot staining technique

TableIII Interpretation of Zhiel results

Number of BAARs	Number of fields examined	Indications
No BAAR	100 fields	0
1 to 9 BAAR	100 fields = 1 length	Exact number
10 to 99 BAAR	100 fields	+
1 to 10 BAAR/Champ	50 fields	++
More than 10 BAAR / Field	20 fields	+++

- The auramine colouring technique

1.2.3.2. Other bacteriological tests

A distinction is made between :

- **So-called phenotypic methods:** culture on solid Löwenstein Jensen medium, on liquid medium such as 7H9 (MGIT 960); and
- **So-called genotyping methods:** rapid diagnostic tests (RDTs) which are molecular methods such as Xpert MTB/RIF available in certain HGR/CSDTs and Hain Life science tests (MDRTB plus or sl) available in certain provincial or central laboratories.

1.2.4. Case definition in the fight against tuberculosis

This section presents the revised definitions of tuberculosis cases, their classification and the categories of therapeutic outcomes.

1.2.4.1. Definitions according to case registration

- **Presumed case of tuberculosis:** Any patient who presents symptoms or signs suggestive of tuberculosis, or who has been infected (previously referred to as a "suspect case", but this stigmatising term is no longer used). (24)

- **Bacteriologically confirmed tuberculosis case (BPT+):** Any patient whose biological sample has been shown to be positive by smear microscopy, culture or WHO-endorsed Rapid Diagnostic Test (RDT) (e.g. Xpert MTB/RIF). These cases should always be notified, whether or not treatment has been started. (24)
- **Clinically diagnosed tuberculosis (cTB):** Any patient who does not meet the criteria for bacteriological confirmation, but in whom the active form has been diagnosed by a clinician or by medical delegation by a trained and regularly supervised healthcare provider. This definition includes cases diagnosed on the basis of suggestive radiographic or histological abnormalities and extra pulmonary cases not confirmed in the laboratory. However, clinically diagnosed cases which are subsequently found to be bacteriologically positive (before or after treatment has been initiated) should be reclassified as bacteriologically confirmed cases. (24)

1.2.4.2. Other types of classification according to registration:

It is important to note that bacteriologically confirmed or clinically diagnosed cases are also classified according to :

- The anatomical site of the disease ;
- Therapeutic history ;
- HIV status ;
- Drug resistance.

a. Classification based on the anatomical site of the disease :

1. **Pulmonary tuberculosis (PT)** refers to any bacteriologically confirmed (PT+) or clinically diagnosed (PT/C) case of tuberculosis in which the lung parenchyma or tracheobronchial tree is affected. Miliary tuberculosis is

considered to be a pulmonary form because it causes lesions in the lungs. (24)

2. **Extrapulmonary tuberculosis (EPT)** refers to any bacteriologically confirmed or clinically diagnosed case of tuberculosis in which organs other than the lungs are involved (e.g. pleura, lymph nodes, abdomen, genitourinary tract, skin, joints and bones, meninges). Intra thoracic tuberculous adenopathy (medial and/or hilar) and tuberculous pleural effusion, without radiographic abnormality of the lungs, are considered to be cases of extra pulmonary tuberculosis. (24)

Extra-pulmonary forms include :

- Extra-pulmonary respiratory tuberculosis, the most common of which is pleurisy;
- Non-respiratory extra-pulmonary tuberculosis includes: lymph node tuberculosis or tuberculous adenitis, pericardial tuberculosis, meningeal tuberculosis, osteoarticular tuberculosis, which can be divided into tuberculosis of the spine or Pott's disease, tuberculosis of the joints, tuberculosis of the long bones, as well as digestive tuberculosis (peritonitis, mesenteric adenitis) and urogenital tuberculosis. (24)

It should be noted that a patient presenting with both a pulmonary and an extra-pulmonary form should be classified as having pulmonary tuberculosis.

b. Classification based on history of anti-tuberculosis treatment.

The classification based on history of anti-tuberculosis treatment differs slightly from that already published. It focuses exclusively on treatment history and is independent of bacteriological confirmation or the site of the disease:

1. **New patients**: are those who have never received anti-tuberculosis treatment or have received it for less than a month.

2. **Previously treated patients**: are those who have received anti-tuberculosis treatment in the past for a period equal to or greater than one month. They are classified according to the therapeutic outcome of their last course of treatment in the following categories:
    - Relapsed patients: are those who have already received anti-tuberculosis treatment, and have been declared cured or treatment completed, and who present a recurrent episode of tuberculosis (relapse as such or new episode due to reinfection).
    - Patients treated after a therapeutic failure: these are patients who have already been treated for tuberculosis and for whom the last course of treatment was inconclusive (therapeutic failure).
    - Patients treated after having been lost to follow-up: these are patients who have already received anti-tuberculosis treatment and have been declared lost to follow-up at the end of their last course of treatment (previously referred to as "patients treated after interruption").
    - Other patients already treated: these are patients who have already received anti-tuberculosis treatment, but for whom the results of the last course of treatment are either unknown or undocumented. (24)
3. **Patients with no known history of anti-tuberculosis treatment** do not fall into any of the above categories.

New patients and relapsed patients are incident cases. Non-relapsed withdrawals are the total of patients treated after a therapeutic failure, patients treated after having been lost to follow-up and other patients already treated.

c. Classification based on drug resistance

Cases are classified into categories on the basis of drug sensitivity tests carried out on confirmed biological isolates of M. tuberculosis:

- ✓ **Mono-resistance**: cases where isolates are resistant to a single first-line anti-tuberculosis drug.
- ✓ **Multi-resistant (MR):** cases in which isolates are resistant to at least isoniazid and rifampicin.
- ✓ **Polyresistance:** cases in which isolates are resistant to more than one first-line anti-tuberculosis drug other than isoniazid and rifampicin.
- ✓ **Ultra resistance (UR):** cases in which isolates are resistant to a fluoroquinolone and to at least one of the three second-line injectable drugs (amikacin, capreomycin and kanamycin), in addition to multi-resistance.
- ✓ **Rifampicin resistance (RR):** cases in which isolates are resistant to rifampicin, detected by phenotypic or genotypic methods, with or without resistance to other anti-tuberculosis drugs. This concept includes all forms of rifampicin resistance (monoresistance, multiresistance, polyresistance or ultraresistance). (24)

A strain is said to be sensitive to the drugs tested when the isolates are sensitive to all the drugs tested. (24)

1.3. Standardised treatment regimens (24)

a) Treatment objectives

The treatment of tuberculosis has the following objectives:

- Healing the sick ;
- To prevent him from dying of tuberculosis or its after-effects;
- Avoiding relapses;
- Reduce the transmission of TB to other people.

b) Essential anti-tuberculosis drugs

a. Isoniazid (INH: isonicotinic acid hydrazide).
b. Rifampicin
c. Pyrazinamide
d. Streptomycin
e. Ethambutol

c) Second-line anti-tuberculosis drugs

1. Aminoglycosides
2. Thioamides :
3. Ciprofloxacin
4. Cycloserine (or Terizidone)
5. Para-aminosalicylic acid (PAS)
6. Others: Rifampicin derivatives (Rifabutin), clofazimine.

d) First-line therapeutic regimens

TableIV First-line therapeutic regimens

Category	Treatment regime	Diagnostics
New patient	2RHZE / 4RH Initial regimen with 1st-line drugs	Bacteriologically confirmed PT
		PD with clinically diagnosed significant or no parenchymal lesions
		Simple or severe PET scans (excluding meningeal, spinal and osteoarticular TB) clinically diagnosed or confirmed
		TB with positive HIV serology and other cases of concomitant severe immunodepression
	2RHZE / 10RH Initial regimen with 1st-line drugs	Severe PET scans: meningeal, spinal and osteoarticular TB
Patient undergoing reprocessing	2SRHZE / RHZE /5RHE Re-treatment regimen with 1st line drugs	Patients in relapse, Patients treated after treatment failure, Patients treated after being lost to follow-up, Other cases already treated.

e) Recording treatment results

At the end of the treatment, the patient is classified in one of the following categories:

- **Cure**: patient giving negative smears at the end, or one month before the end of treatment, as well as another time before this last examination.

- **Complete treatment**: patient who has completed treatment but for whom sputum smear results are not available on at least two occasions before the end of treatment.
- **Failure**: patient still giving positive smears or giving positive smears again after five months or more of treatment.
- **Death**: patient who dies during treatment, whatever the reason for death.
- **Treatment interrupted** (discontinuation): patient who has interrupted treatment for two months or more.
- **Transfer**: patient transferred to another care unit for whom the outcome of the treatment is unknown.

Chapter II: MATERIALS AND METHODS

II.1 Research framework

Our study took place in Kisangani, the capital of Tshopo province in the Democratic Republic of Congo. This city has 20 Tuberculosis Diagnostic and Treatment Centres (CDT), and we chose 3 of them because they were much more frequented. These are :

- CDT SAINT JOSEPH
- CDT IMANI
- THE MILITARY HOSPITAL

II.2 Equipment

II.2.1. Population

Our study population consisted of 191 tuberculosis patients (all forms combined) diagnosed and treated in the above-mentioned CDTs during our study period, who were 15 years of age or older.

II.2.2. Sample

We used convenience sampling. The minimum sample size was calculated using GPower software version 3.1.9.7 and was 143 individuals. Based on our inclusion and exclusion criteria, our sample consisted of 171 patients.

Inclusion criteria

- All cases of tuberculosis diagnosed and treated in the CDTs in our study.
- Be at least 15 years old
- Have given informed consent

Exclusion criteria

All cases of :

- Discontinuation of treatment ;
- Transfer to another structure

II.2.5. Flow diagram.

We enrolled 191 patients in our study, 20 of whom were excluded from the study, including 6 who discontinued treatment and 14 who were transferred to other facilities.

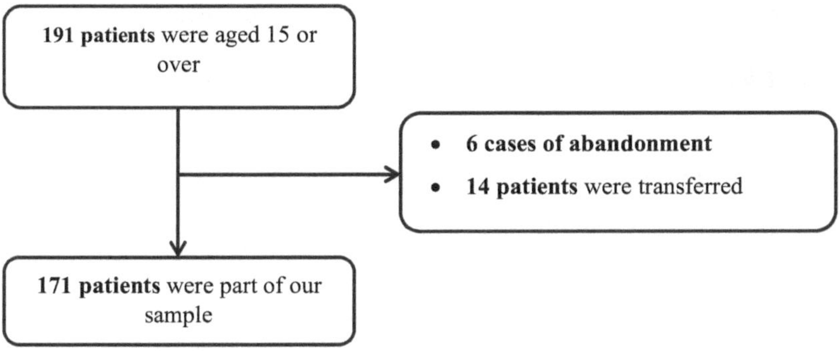

Figure1 : Flow chart

II.3 Methods

II.3.1. Type and period of study

This is a prospective cohort study. The study covers the period from 01 July 2022 to 31 December 2022 for the recruitment period. The follow-up period was until 31 March 2023, as the intensive phase lasts 3 months for patients undergoing retreatment.

II.3.2. Data collection

Each patient was monitored for at least 2 months (2 months for new cases and 3 months for patients already treated) and seen once a month.

II.3.2.1. Data sources

The information was gathered by :

- Interviewing patients during diagnosis
- On consultation forms for tuberculosis patients
- Patient medical records
- Patient treatment forms

- The laboratory register
- Patient follow-up register
- The follow-up register for PLWHA-TB patients

II.3.2.1. Study variables

The information gathered by interviewing patients was as follows:

- **Identity:** name and surname, age, sex, marital status, profession, religion, employer and address;
- **Housing conditions**: Type of house, type of flooring, number of people in the room, size of the room, location of the kitchen, type of fuel used, type of toilet;
- **The person funding the treatment ;**
- **The history of the disease:** the date of onset of the first symptoms, the patient's history prior to diagnosis, the health facilities consulted;
- **Medical history:** history of contagious diseases, smoking, alcoholism, diabetes, gout, HIV, heart disease, high blood pressure.
- **Clinical manifestations**

We collected the following data from the files, consultation forms, treatment forms and follow-up registers for tuberculosis patients and the follow-up register for PLWHA-TB:

- Clinical manifestations
- Treatment received: anti-tuberculosis treatment, ARV treatment if the patient was co-infected with HIV-TB
- Compliance with treatment
- Progression under treatment
- Radiological signs
- The form of tuberculosis
- End of treatment at the end of the intensive phase.

The following data were collected in the laboratory register:

- **Paraclinical tests:** Zhiel result, Genexpert, HIV serology,

II.3.4. Operational definitions

- **Survivor :** Patient alive at the end of the intensive anti-tuberculosis treatment phase.
- **Death**: Patient died of tuberculosis during the intensive treatment phase.
- **Treatment interrupted (discontinuation)**: Patient who has interrupted treatment and has not been found by the community relay for a month or more.
- **Transfer**: Patient transferred to another care unit for whom the outcome of the treatment is unknown. (26)
- **DOT or TDO** (Directly Observed Treatment): This is when taking medication is supervised by a trained and supervised health worker or community relay or a trained family member. (26)
- **Compliance:** The fact of regularly taking at least 85% of the treatment, at the indicated time and in the indicated doses.
- **Consultation period:** This is the interval between the start date of the first events and the date of the first consultation at the CDT.
- **Profound alteration of general condition:** This syndrome is characterised by weight loss of more than 10%, anorexia, intense physical asthenia and bed rest.
- **New case*:* *a*** patient who has never received anti-tuberculosis treatment or who has taken anti-tuberculosis drugs for less than four weeks.
- **Previously treated cases:** patients who have previously received anti-tuberculosis treatment for at least one month.

II.3.5. Data processing and analysis techniques

Data were entered on a computer using Microsoft Excel 2016. Statistical analysis of the data was carried out using R software version 4.2.3.

We used percentage and mean calculations. We used the chi-square test and Fisher's exact test to compare proportions, and the Mann-Whitney U test to compare means.

To identify risk factors for death in the intensive phase, we calculated crude relative risk using univariate logistic regression and adjusted relative risk using multivariate logistic regression. The statistical significance threshold was 0.05 and the confidence interval was 95%. The results were presented in tabular form.

II.5. Difficulties encountered

We encountered a number of difficulties, including

- Given that the study was prospective, it was very expensive;
- The collection of data was very laborious;
- Some of our patients had gone missing.

II.6. Ethical considerations

This study complied with the standards of the National Tuberculosis Control Programme (PNLT) and the National AIDS Control Programme (PNLS). All data accessible during the study were kept confidential and no disclosure was made of patients' names or serostatus. All patients who participated in our study signed a consent form.

Chapter III: RESULTS

3.1. Socio-demographic characteristics

The table shows the socio-demographic characteristics of our patients. These include age, sex, marital status, level of education, occupation and religion.

Our patients ranged in age from 15 to 84 years, with an average age of 40.41 ± 17.64 years.

Table VV Socio-demographic characteristics

Socio-demographic characteristics	N = 171	p-value
Age in years		0,02
15 to 35 years old	79 (46%)	
36 - 55 years old	55 (32%)	
> 55 years	37 (22%)	
Gender		0,003
Female	61 (36%)	
Male	110 (64%)	
Level of study		< 0,0001
Primary	19 (11%)	
Secondary	98 (57%)	
University	54 (32%)	
Civil status		< 0,0001
Single	51 (30%)	
Divorced	1 (0,6%)	
Married	111 (65%)	
Widow(er)	8 (4,7%)	
Municipality		< 0,0001
Tshopo	96 (56%)	
Makiso	60 (35%)	
Mangobo	7 (4,1%)	
Kabondo	5 (2,9%)	
Out of town	2 (1,2%)	
Kisangani	1 (0,6%)	
Profession		0,6
Formal sector	87 (51%)	
Informal sector	84 (49%)	
Religion		< 0,0001
Church of revival	78 (46%)	
Catholic	60 (35%)	
Protestant	21 (12%)	
Muslim	9 (5,3%)	
Kimbaguiste	3 (1,8%)	

Table V shows that :

- The most represented age group was between 15 and 35 (46%);
- Men were the most represented, with a frequency of 64%;
- Subjects with secondary education were the most represented (57%);
- Married people were the most represented (65%);

- The majority of our respondents lived in the commune of Tshopo (56%);
- Subjects from the formal sector were the most represented (51%);
- Christians from revivalist churches were the most represented at 46%.

3.2. Forms of tuberculosis

The following table shows the distribution of tuberculosis patients according to the clinical form of the disease.

TableVI Breakdown of cases by type of tuberculosis

Forms of tuberculosis	N = 171	p-value
Pulmonary tuberculosis		< 0,0001
TP+	128 (75%)	
TP/C	29 (17%)	
Extra pulmonary tuberculosis		
Pleuresis	10 (5,8%)	
Ganglion	1 (0,6%)	
Peritonitis	1 (0,6%)	
Bone	1 (0,6%)	
Cutaneous	1 (0,6%)	

This table shows that bacilloscopy-positive pulmonary tuberculosis is the most represented clinical form (75%), followed by clinically diagnosed pulmonary tuberculosis (17%). In total, pulmonary tuberculosis was the most common form, accounting for 91% of cases.

3.3. HIV serology

Table VII shows the distribution of cases according to HIV serology.

TableVII Distribution of cases according to HIV serology

HIV serology	N = 171	p-value
Negative	73 (43%)	< 0,0001
Positive	20 (12%)	
Not carried out	78 (46%)	

This table shows that 46% of our patients had not undergone HIV serology and 12% of our patients were seropositive.

3.4. Mortality in the intensive phase of treatment

Of the 171 patients in our study, 19 died during the intensive phase, giving a mortality rate of 11.11%. The total survival time of our patients was 331.56 person-months. The mortality risk was 57.3 deaths per 1000 person-months.

Table VIII below shows the timing of 19 deaths in weeks:

TableVIII Mortality trends over time

Week	N = 19	Cumulative
1st Week	7 (37%)	37
Week 2	5 (26%)	63
3rd week	3 (16%)	79
4th week	0 (0%)	79
5th week	2 (11%)	90
6th week	1 (5%)	95
8th week	1 (5%)	100

The table shows that 37% of deaths occurred in the first week, 26% in the second week and 16% in the third week. The majority of deaths, 79%, occurred in the first month.

3.5. Socio-demographic characteristics and mortality

In our study, we had 152 survivors and 19 deaths at the end of the intensive anti-tuberculosis treatment phase. Among the survivors, the age limits were 15 years and 85 years with an average of 38.8 ±16.3. In contrast, the age limits for deceased subjects were 18 years and 78 years, with an average of 53.7± 22.5 years. Comparison of these 2 averages shows a statistically significant difference ($p = 0.006$ with the non-parametric Mann-Whitney test).

Table VI below shows the associations between the socio-demographic characteristics of subjects and death during the intensive phase of anti-tuberculosis treatment.

TableIX Socio-demographic characteristics and risk factors for death of respondents

Socio-demographic characteristics	WORKFORCE N = 171	Deaths (n = 19, (%))	RR	95% CI	p-value
Age in years					
15 to 35 years old	79	6 (7,6%)	0,54	0,32 - 1,47	0,5
36 - 55 years old	55	1 (1,8%)	0,12	0,01 - 1,32	0,2
> 55 years	37	12 (32,4%)	6,21	1,74 - 12,4	**0,003**
Gender					
Female	61	9 (14,8%)	1,62	0,28 - 6,42	0,7
Male	110	10 (9,1%)	0,62	0,26 - 1,48	0,3
Level of study					
University	54	3 (5,6%)	0,41	0,12 - 1,27	0,09
Primary	19	6 (31,6%)	3,69	1,54 - 20,3	**0,021**
Secondary	98	10 (10,2%)	0,83	0,59 - 7,52	0,5
Civil status					
Single	51	6 (11,8%)	1,09	0,54 - 3,44	0,2
Divorced	1	0 (0,0%)	0	0.00 - Inf	>0,9
Married	111	10 (9,0%)	0,6	0,29 - 2,02	0,6
Widower	8	3 (37,5%)	3,82	0,85 - 12,0	0,085
Municipality					
Kabondo	5	0 (0,0%)	0	0.00 - Inf	>0,9
Kisangani	1	0 (0,0%)	0	0.00 - Inf	>0,9
Makiso	60	6 (10,0%)	0,85	0,34 - 2,45	0,8
Mangobo	7	1 (14,3%)	1,30	0,64 - 3,53	0,7
Periphery	2	0 (0,0%)	0	0.00 - Inf	>0,9
Tshopo	96	12 (12,5%)	1,34	0,58 - 3,58	0,6
Profession					
Formal sector	87	5 (5,7%)	0,31	0,12 - 0,72	**0,012**
Informal sector	84	14 (16,7%)	2,9	1,16 - 8,41	**0,033**
Religion					

Catholic	60	6 (10,0%)	0,85	0,34 - 2,32	0,6
Church of revival	78	7 (9,0%)	0,7	0,39 - 2,64	0,8
Kimbaguiste	3	0 (0,0%)	0	0.00 - Inf	>0,9
Muslim	9	3 (33,3%)	3,33	0,89 - 12,5	0,072
Protestant	21	3 (14,3%)	1,43	0,38 - 5,36	0,6

3.5.1. Age and mortality

Table IX shows that mortality occurs at all ages, but the risk of death was higher when the patient was aged 55 or over (RR=6.21 95% CI: 1.74 - 12.4 p=0.003).

3.5.2. Gender and mortality

In our study, mortality was higher in women than in men, but the difference was not statistically significant (RR=1.62 95% CI: 0.28 - 6.42 p=0.7).

3.5.3. Level of education

Table IX shows that subjects with all levels of education were affected by mortality, but patients with primary education were the most exposed to death (RR=3.69 95% CI: 1.54 - 20.3 p=0.021).

3.5.4. Marital status and mortality

Widowers had the highest mortality among those most affected, with 3 deaths out of 8 patients, followed by bachelors (11%), but the difference was not statistically significant (RR= 3.88, 95% CI: 0.85 - 12.0 p= 0.085).

3.5.5. Municipality of residence and mortality

Mortality was higher in Mangobo commune with 1 death out of 7 patients, i.e. 14% (RR= 1.73 95% CI: 0.74 - 8.53 p=0.7), followed by Tshopo commune with 12 deaths out of 96 patients, i.e. 12% (RR= 1.34 95% CI: 0.58 - 3.58 p=0.6). However, the difference was not statistically significant.

3.5.6. Occupations and mortality

The risk of death was higher when the patient was in the informal sector (RR=2.9 95% CI: 1.16 - 8.41 p=0.033).

3.5.7. Religion and mortality during the intensive phase

Mortality was higher among Muslims, i.e. 3 out of 9 subjects (33.3%) (RR= 3.33 95% CI: 0.89 - 12.5 p=0.072). The differences observed between religions were not statistically significant.

3.6. History of the disease, co-morbidity and mortality

The table below shows the association between antecedents, history of illness and death during the intensive phase of anti-tuberculosis treatment.

Table XX Association of antecedents and death during the intensive phase

History	WORKFORCE N = 171	Deaths (n = 19, (%))	RR	95% CI	p-value
Notion of tuberculosis infection					
No	127	17 (13,4%)	2,94	0,65 - 5,62	0,4
Yes	44	2 (4,5%)	0,34	0,05 - 1,18	0,15
Notion of smoking					
No	135	9 (6,7%)	0,24	0,02 - 0,89	**0,003**
Yes	36	10 (27,8%)	4,17	1,68 - 10,5	**0,002**
Notion of alcoholism					
No	99	6 (6,1%)	0,34	0,08 - 0,89	**0,04**
Yes	72	13 (18,1%)	2,98	1,18 - 8,48	**0,027**
Diabetes mellitus					
No	154	15 (9,7%)	0,41	0,07 - 2,45	0,2
Yes	17	4 (23,5%)	2,42	0,69 - 6,66	0,12
Drop					
No	169	19 (11,2%)	Inf	0.00 - Inf	>0,9
Yes	2	0 (0,0%)	0	0.00 - Inf	>0,9
Bronchial asthma					
No	167	16 (9,6%)	0,13	0,04 - 0,52	**0,002**
Yes	4	3 (75,0%)	7,83	1,82 - 23,5	**0,001**
Heart disease					
No	164	17 (10,4%)	0,36	0,14 - 2,61	0,6
Yes	7	2 (28,6%)	2,76	0,44 - 9,61	0,2
Sickle cell disease					
No	166	18 (10,8%)	0,54	0,26 - 3,65	0,7
Yes	5	1 (20,0%)	1,84	0,10 - 8,93	0,6
Consultation period					
≤ 30 days	15	1 (6,7%)	0,58	0,03 - 0,90	**0,046**
> 30 days	156	18 (11,5%)	1,73	1,04 - 5,26	**0,045**
HIV serology					
Negative	73	7 (9,6%)	0,78	0,44 - 1,64	0,5
Positive	20	10 (50,0%)	5,21	2,00 - 14,4	**<0,001**
Not carried out	78	2 (2,6%)	0,27	0,04 - 1,11	0,1

3.7.1. Notion of tuberculosis infection

According to Table X, the existence of a contact is not associated with tuberculosis (RR = 0.34, 95% CI: 0.05 - 1.18; p = 0.15).

3.7.2. Notion of smoking

In our study, subjects who knew they smoked were the most likely to die (RR = 4.17; 95% CI: 1.68 - 10.5; p = 0.002).

3.7.3. Notion of alcoholism

Table X shows that alcoholics were more likely to die than non-alcoholics (RR = 2.98; 95% CI = 1.18 - 8.48; p = 0.027).

3.7.4. Diabetes mellitus

According to Table X, a history of diabetes mellitus was not associated with mortality (RR = 2.42; 95% CI: 0.69 - 6.66; p = 0.12).

3.7.5. Drop

In our study, a history of diabetes mellitus was not associated with mortality (RR = 0; 95% CI: 0.00 - Inf; p > 0.9).

3.7.6. Bronchial asthma

In our study, subjects with a history of asthma were more exposed than those without (RR = .7.83; 95% CI: 1.82 - 23.5; p = 0.001).

3.7.7. Heart disease

Table X shows that previous heart disease was not associated with mortality (RR = 2.76; 95% CI: 0.44 - 9.6; p = 0.2).

3.7.8. Sickle cell disease

In the preceding table (Table X), a history of sickle cell disease was not associated with mortality (RR = 1.84; 95% CI: 0.10 - 8.93; p = 0.6).

3.7.9. Consultation period

In Table X, subjects who had consulted within more than 1 month were more exposed than those who had consulted within ≤ 30 days (RR = .1.73; 95% CI: 1.04 - 5.26; p = 0.046).

The mean time to consultation was 56 days for those who survived, compared with 76 days for those who died; the minimum and maximum times were 26 and 120 days respectively for those who survived, and 30 and 150 days respectively for those who died. The difference was statistically significant using the Wilcoxon-Mann-Whitney test (p = 0.0032).

3.7.10. HIV serology and death in the intensive phase

Table X shows that HIV-positive subjects were more likely to die during the intensive phase of TB treatment (RR = 5.21; CI =2.00 - 14.4; p <0.001).

3.8. Clinical aspects

3.8.1. Respiratory symptoms and mortality

Table XI shows the association between respiratory symptoms and death during the intensive phase of tuberculosis treatment.

TableXI Measure of association between respiratory symptoms and death

Respiratory symptoms	WORKFORCE N = 171	Deaths (n = 19, (%))	RR	95% CI	p-value
Cough					
No cough	6	1 (16,7%)	1,53	0,55 - 6,53	0,5
Cough < 1 month	19	0 (0,0%)	0	0.00 - Inf	>0,9
Cough ≥ 1 month	146	18 (12,3%)	3,08	0,10 - 5,54	0,8
Dyspnoea					
No	111	6 (5,4%)	0,25	0,15 - 0,74	**0,003**
Yes	60	13 (21,7%)	4,01	1,58 - 11,4	**0,005**
Sputum					
No	21	2 (9,5%)	0,84	0,24 - 6,54	0,6
Yes	150	17 (11,3%)	1,19	0,34 - 7,51	0,8
Haemoptysis					
No	149	10 (6,7%)	0,16	0,05 - 0,67	**0,003**
Yes	22	9 (40,9%)	6,1	2,42 - 15,1	**<0,001**
Chest pain					
No	62	4 (6,5%)	0,47	0,17 - 2,53	0,5
Yes	109	15 (13,8%)	2,13	0,77 - 7,48	0,2

3.8.1.1. Cough

According to the table above, cough is not associated with death in the intensive phase of tuberculosis treatment (RR= 3.08; 95% CI: 0.10 - 5.54; p = 0.8).

3.8.1.2. Dyspnoea

Table XI shows that subjects with dyspnoea were more likely to die during the intensive phase of TB treatment than those without dyspnoea (RR = 4.01; 95% CI: 1.58 - 11.4 p = 0.005).

3.8.1.3. Expectorations

In our study, there was no association between sputum and death in the intensive phase of TB treatment (RR = 1.19; 95% CI: 0.34 - 7.51; p = 0.8).

3.8.1.4. Haemoptysis

According to Table XI, subjects with haemoptysis were more likely to die in the intensive phase of treatment than those without (RR = 6.1 95% CI: 2.42 - 15.1; $p < 0.001$).

3.8.1.5. Chest pain

In our study, there was no association between chest pain and death in the intensive phase of TB treatment (RR = 2.13; 95% CI: 0.77 - 7.48; $p = 0.2$).

3.8.2. Non-respiratory signs and mortality

Table XII below shows the association between non-respiratory signs and death in the intensive phase.

TableXII Measure of association between non-respiratory signs and death in the intensive phase of tuberculosis treatment.

Non-respiratory signs	**WORKFORCE** N = 171	**Deaths** (n = 19, (%))	**RR**	**95% CI**	**p-value**
Fever					
No	1	0 (0,0%)	0	0.00 - Inf	>0,9
Yes	170	19 (11,2%)	494 462	0.00 - Inf	>0,9
Physical asthenia					
No	42	3 (7,1%)	0,58	0,34 - 3,56	0,5
Yes	129	16 (12,4%)	1,74	0,61 - 6,83	0,4
Weight loss					
No	9	0 (0,0%)	0	0.00 - Inf	>0,9
Yes	162	19 (11,7%)	Inf	0.00 - Inf	>0,9
Night sweats					
No	9	0 (0,0%)	0	0.00 - Inf	>0,9
Yes	162	19 (11,7%)	Inf	0.00 - Inf	>0,9
Vertigo					
No	136	6 (4,4%)	0,12	0,03 - 0,54	**<0,001**
Yes	35	13 (37,1%)	8,42	3,49 - 22,6	**<0,001**
Diarrhoea					
No	153	18 (11,8%)	2,12	0,53 - 6,27	0,5
Yes	18	1 (5,6%)	0,47	0,03 - 2,14	0,4
Pallor					
No	153	9 (5,9%)	0,11	0,02 - 0,57	**<0,001**
Yes	18	10 (55,6%)	9,44	3,99 - 22,6	**<0,001**
Attitude					
Ambulante	151	8 (5,3%)	0,1	0,02 - 0,55	**<0,001**
Bedridden	20	11 (55,0%)	10,4	4,40 - 25,5	**<0,001**
Profound deterioration in general condition					
No	148	7 (4,7%)	0,09	0,01 - 0,56	**<0,001**
Yes	23	12 (52,2%)	11	4,65 - 28,1	**<0,001**
Adenopathies					
No	119	12 (10,1%)	0,75	0,34 - 3,76	0,6
Yes	52	7 (13,5%)	1,33	0,52 - 3,17	0,5
BMI					
$\geq$ 18.5 kg/m^2	84	5 (6,0%)	0,37	0,23 - 0,82	**0,045**
< 18.5 kg/m^2	87	14 (16,1%)	2,7	1,08 - 7,84	**0,046**

The table shows that fever, physical asthenia, weight loss, night sweats, diarrhoea, the presence of adenopathies and ascites are not associated with mortality in the intensive phase.

However, the following factors were associated with mortality:

- Vertigo (RR = 8.42; CI = 3.49 - 22.6; $p < 0.001$);
- Pallor (RR = 9.44; CI = 3.99 - 22.6; $p < 0.001$);
- Bedridden attitude (RR = 10.4; CI = 4.40 - 25.5; $p < 0.001$);
- Profound impairment of general condition (RR = 11; CI = 4.65 - 28.1; $p < 0.001$) and
- BMI <18.5 $kg/m^{(2)}$ (RR = 2.7; CI = 1.08 - 7.84; $p = 0.46$).

The mean BMI was 18.7 $kg/m^2$for those who survived compared with 16.7 $kg/m^2$for those who died; the minimum and maximum BMIs were 13.7 and 27.1 kg/m^2respectively for those who survived and 13.6 and 24.3 $kg/m^{(2)}$) respectively for those who died. The difference was statistically significant using the non-parametric Wilcoxon-Manny-Whitney test ($p<0.001$).

3.9. Forms of tuberculosis and mortality

In our study, we had 153 cases of PT, 10 cases of pleurisy and 8 cases of non-thoracic PET. Of these 8 cases of non-thoracic PET, we did not record any deaths. Table XIII below shows the association between the different forms of thoracic tuberculosis and mortality during the intensive phase of tuberculosis treatment.

Table XIIIXIII Association between forms of tuberculosis and mortality in the intensive phase.

Thoracic tuberculosis	WORKFORCE N = 163	Deaths (n = 19, (%))	RR	95% CI	p-value
TP+	128	15 (11,7%)	1,26	0,34 - 3,46	0,7
TP/C	25	3 (12,0%)	1,1	0,30 - 3,54	0,6
Pleuresis	10	1 (10,0%)	0,89	0,11 - 6,46	0,9

This table shows that there was no association between the clinical forms of tuberculosis and death in the intensive phase ($p > 0.9$).

3.10. Treatment category and mortality in the intensive phase

Table XVI shows the association between treatment categories, side-effects and mortality in the intensive phase of tuberculosis.

Table XIVXIV Association between treatment category and mortality in the intensive phase

Variables	WORKFORCE N = 171	Deaths (n = 19, (%))	RR	95% CI	p-value
Treatment category					
New case	164	18 (11,0%)	0,77	0,57 - 2,52	0,5
Case already dealt with	7	1 (14,3%)	1,3	0,07 - 6,30	0,8

This table shows that the category of treatment and side effects are not associated with death in the intensive phase of tuberculosis treatment.

3.11. Risk factors for mortality in the intensive phase of tuberculosis

After univariate analysis, the following factors showed a statistically significant association with mortality in the intensive phase of anti-tuberculosis treatment:

- Age > 55 (RR=6.21 95% CI: 1.74 - 12.4 p=0.003);
- Level of primary education (RR=3.69 95% CI: 1.54 - 20.3 p=0.021);
- Being in the informal sector (RR=2.9 95% CI: 1.16 - 8.41 p=0.033) ;
- Time to consultation.> 30 days ((RR = .1.73; 95% CI: 1.04 - 5.26; p = 0.046) ;
- Smoking habits (RR = 4.17; 95% CI: 1.68 - 10.5; p = 0.002);
- Alcoholism (RR = 2.98; 95% CI = 1.18 - 8.48; p = 0.027);
- Asthma (RR = .7.83; 95% CI: 1.82 - 23.5; p = 0.001);
- Dyspnoea (RR = 4.01; 95% CI: 1.58 - 11.4 p = 0.005);
- Haemoptysis (RR = 6.1 95% CI: 2.42 - 15.1; p <0.001);
- Pallor (RR = 9.44; CI = 3.99 - 22.6; p <0.001);

- Vertigo (RR = 8.42; CI = 3.49 - 22.6; p <0.001);
- Bedridden attitude (RR = 10.4; CI = 4.40 - 25.5; p < 0.001);
- Profound deterioration in general condition (RR 11; CI = 4.65 - 28.1; p < 0.001)
- Positive HIV serology (RR = 5.21; CI =2.00 - 14.4; p <0.001) and
- BMI < 18.5 kg/$m^{(2)}$ (RR = 2.7; CI = 1.08 - 7.84; p = 0.046).

We therefore performed multivariate analysis by logistic regression with these variables in order to determine the best predictors or risk factors for mortality in the intensive phase of tuberculosis treatment.

Table XVII presents the results of multivariate analyses by logistic regression of the various factors whose association with death was statistically significant.

TableXV Univariate and multivariate analyses

Variables	WORKFORCE N = 171	Deaths (n = 19, (%))	Multivariate analysis		
			RR[2]	95% IC[2]	p-value
Age in years					
15 to 35 years old	79	6 (7,6%)	Ref	-	
36 - 55 years old	55	1 (1,8%)	0,13	0,03 - 1,60	0,08
> 55 years	37	12 (32,4%)	**3,39**	1,57 - 13,36	**0,005**
Level of study					
University	54	3 (5,6%)	Ref	-	
Primary	19	6 (31,6%)	0,96	0,10 - 9,40	>0,9
Secondary	98	10 (10,2%)	2,74	0,91 - 8,30	0,071
Profession					
Employees	87	5 (5,7%)	Ref	-	
Non-employees	84	14 (16,7%)	5,18	2,03 - 13,2	**<0,001**
Consultation period					
> 30 days	156	18 (11,5%)	Ref	-	
≤ 30 days	15	1 (6,7%)	0,43	0,22 - 0,88	**0,036**
Notion of smoking					
No	135	9 (6,7%)	Ref	-	
Yes	36	10 (27,8%)	2,38	1,51 -13,75	**0,025**
Notion of alcoholism					
No	99	6 (6,1%)	Ref	-	
Yes	72	13 (18,1%)	**2,22**	1,50 - 12,99	**0,017**
Asthma					
No	167	16 (9,6%)	Ref	-	
Yes	4	3 (75,0%)	0,95	0,32 - 2,83	>0,9
Dyspnoea					
No	111	6 (5,4%)	Ref	-	
Yes	60	13 (21,7%)	1,92	1,84 - 6,41	0,012
Haemoptysis					
No	149	10 (6,7%)	Ref	-	
Yes	22	9 (40,9%)	0,6	0,24 - 1,50	0,3

Variables	WORKFORCE N = 171	Deaths (n = 19, (%))	Multivariate analysis		
			RR[2]	95% IC[2]	p-value
Pallor					
No	153	9 (5,9%)	Ref	-	
Yes	18	10 (55,6%)	2,41	1,51 - 8,35	**0,027**
Vertigo					
No	136	6 (4,4%)	Ref	-	
Yes	35	13 (37,1%)	2,32	1,42 - 14,12	**0,036**
Attitude					
Ambulante	151	8 (5,3%)	Ref	-	
Bedridden	20	11 (55,0%)	1,7	1,43 - 13,15	**0,028**
Profound deterioration in general condition					
No	148	7 (4,7%)	Ref	-	
Yes	23	12 (52,2%)	3,01	1,42 - 6,38	**0,004**
Serology					
Negative	73	7 (9,6%)	Ref	-	
Not carried out	78	2 (2,6%)	0,21	0,07 - 1,63	0,054
Positive	20	10 (50,0%)	3,62	1,21 - 11,85	**0,004**
BMI					
≥ 18.5 kg/m²	84	5 (6,0%)	Ref	-	
< 18.5 kg/m²	87	14 (16,1%)	**2,08**	1,46 - 5,55	**0,039**

3.11.9. Multivariate analysis

After multivariate analysis, the following factors showed a statistically significant association with mortality in the intensive treatment phase:

- Age > 55 (RR = 3.39; CI = 1.57 - 13.36; p = 0.005);
- Being self-employed (RR=2.9; 95% CI: 2.03 - 13.2, p=0.001);
- Smoking (RR = 2.38; CI = 1.51 -13.75; p = 0.025);
- Alcoholism (RR = 2.22; CI = 1.50 - 12.99; p = 0.017);
- Consultation time ≤ 30 days (RR = 0.43; CI = 0.22 - 0.88; p = 0.036);
- Dyspnoea (RR = 1.92; CI = 1.84 - 6.41; p = 0.012);
- Pallor (RR = 2.41; CI = 1.51 - 8.35; p = 0.027);

- Vertigo (RR = 2.32; CI = 1.42 - 14.12; p = 0.036);
- Bedridden attitude (RR = 1.7; CI = 1.43 - 13.15; p = 0.028);
- Profound deterioration in general condition (RR = 3.01; CI = 1.42 - 6.38; p = 0.004);
- HIV-positive serology (RR = 3.62; CI = 1.21 - 11.85; p = 0.004) and
- BMI < 18.5 kg/m$^{(2)}$ (RR = 2.08; CI = 1.46 - 1.55; p = 0.039).

Chapter IV: DISCUSSION

4.1. Mortality in the intensive phase

In our study, of the 171 patients followed up, 19 died during the intensive phase, giving a mortality rate of 11.11%. The mortality risk was 57.3 deaths per 1000 person-months.

The mortality found in our study is higher than that found by Osman Abdullahi et al, in Kenya in 2019 (7.2%) (6) . In the study conducted by Adamu AL et al, in Nigeria in 2017, mortality was 16.6%(7) . Although these studies were conducted over the entire duration of tuberculosis treatment, the majority of these deaths occurred during the intensive treatment phase in the first few months of treatment. These results show that mortality during the intensive phase of tuberculosis treatment is still very high in sub-Saharan Africa. This excess mortality here can be explained by the fact that most of our patients arrived late and at an advanced stage of the disease. (See table X)

As for the timing of this mortality, 79% of all deaths occurred in the first month (see Table VIII). These results are similar to those of Adamu et al who found that approximately half of the deaths occurred during the first week of treatment and that approximately three quarters of deaths occurred during the first month. Early death and clinical worsening after treatment initiation were associated with drug toxicity and comorbidities in studies conducted by Waitt CJ et al(27) , in 2011, Bisson GP et al(28) , in 2015, Pepper DJ et al(29) , in South Africa in 2009, and Gupta A et al(30) in 2011.

4.2 Factors associated with mortality during the intensive phase of treatment

In our study we identified the following as risk factors for mortality in the intensive phase of tuberculosis treatment: age > 55 years, consultation > 30 days, smoking, alcoholism, a history of HIV, dyspnoea, pallor, dizziness, bed rest, profound deterioration in general condition, positive HIV serology, hospitalisation at the CDT and BMI < 18.5, all of which were associated with death in the univariate and multivariate analyses (see Table XV).

Other mortality risk factors such as primary education, asthma and haemoptysis were not associated with death in the multivariate analysis (see Table XV).

4.2.1. Age

In our study, subjects aged over 55 years were 3.39 times more likely to die during the intensive phase of treatment than subjects aged between 15 and 35 years (RR = 3.39, CI = 1.57 - 13.36; p = 0.005). (See table XV)

Peter Seah Keng TokIP et al(31) , in a study of risk factors for mortality during tuberculosis treatment in Malaysia in 2020, found that the risk of dying from tuberculosis increases with age. They showed that from the age of 12, each additional year increases the risk of dying by 1,039 (CI: 1,037 - 1,040). Adil Sbadyi et al, in Morocco in 2020, found by comparing ages that death occurred preferentially in older subjects. In this study, subjects aged 50 to 59 were 2 times more likely to die than young people aged 20 to 29, and subjects aged 70 and over were 6 times more likely to die than subjects aged 20 to 29(20) . Osman A. AbdullahiI et al, in their study in Kenya in 2019, found that subjects aged over 45 were 3.8 times more likely to die than young people under 15 and 1.4 times more likely to die than subjects aged between 15 and 45. In the study conducted by Muhammad Osman et al in South Africa in 2021, subjects aged 65 and over had a 5.22-fold greater risk of dying than subjects aged 15 to 24 (CI: 5.1-5.33) . (21)

The explanation we can give for this is that tuberculosis is a disease in which the risk of death increases as the immune defence system declines(26) . With immunosenescence, as age advances, the immune system weakens and the risk of dying during treatment for tuberculosis increases. The high risk of mortality in elderly subjects could also be explained by the ageing of systems and the association of several co-morbidities that occur with age.

4.2.2. Level of study

Univariate analyses showed that subjects with a primary level of education were 5.68 times more likely to die in the intensive phase of TB treatment than university graduates (CI = 1.60 - 24.7; p = 0.011). However, multivariate analyses did not show a statistically significant association between level of education and death. (See table XV)

Peter Seah Keng Tok et al(31) found in their series that there was a statistically significant association between levels of education and death during tuberculosis treatment. In this study, the higher the level of education, the lower the risk of death. In other words, subjects with no formal education were more exposed than those with primary education; the latter were more exposed than those with secondary education, and so on.

This can be explained by the fact that the more educated the subjects, the more readily they go to hospital for treatment. The less educated they are, the more they rely on traditional medicines and spend too much time before going to hospital. The relationship between level of education and poverty attests to the idea that education improves household living standards. In France, according to INSEE data for 2019, 80% of poor people have not gone beyond the baccalauréat, and almost 30% have no qualifications at all. The poverty rate is 2.4 times higher for non-graduates (11.1%) than for graduates with 3 or more years of higher education (4.6%). In terms of numbers, poor people without qualifications (1.1 million) are 2.6 times more numerous than the 432,000 poor people with a degree or higher(32) . In the DRC, analysis by the African Development Bank in 2010 showed that households with a low level of education are the most exposed to poverty, with 76% compared with only 34% for households with a university or post-graduate level of education(33) . The fact that tuberculosis is a disease linked to poverty would justify the high frequency of cases among people with a low level of education.

4.2.3. Profession or occupation

In our study, non-employees were 5.18 times more likely to die than employees. (See table XV)

Our results differ from those of K. Adjoh et al, who found in a study carried out in 2016 on factors associated with death among tuberculosis patients in the intensive phase of treatment at the Sylvanus Olympio University Hospital in Lomé that employees were 3 times more exposed (OR = 3.0267) .(34)

We believe that the increase in mortality among the self-employed is due to the fact that the majority of people without a salary in the DRC are often not in a position to look after themselves in the event of illness, which means that they often arrive in hospital at an advanced stage of the disease.

4.2.3. Notion of smoking

In our study, subjects who smoked were 2.38 times more likely to die during the intensive phase of tuberculosis treatment than non-smokers (CI = 1.51 -13.75; p = 0.025). (See table XV)

Peter Seah Keng Tok et al, demonstrated in their study that there is a statistically significant relationship between mortality during tuberculosis treatment and smoking(31) . This study showed that smokers have a higher risk of death than non-smokers. Antoine D et al also demonstrated in their studies that smoking is significantly associated with death during tuberculosis treatment(35) . Bulckaen H et al also made the same finding .(36)

Tobacco contains substances (nicotine, tar, etc) that are harmful to the body, leading to slow, gradual destruction of the lungs and their defence mechanisms. Tobacco not only affects the diseased lungs of tuberculosis patients, but can also have a negative impact on anti-tuberculosis treatment and reduce the effectiveness of the drugs. (26)

4.2.4. Notion of alcoholism

Our study showed that patients with a history of alcoholism were 2.22 times more likely to die in the intensive phase of TB treatment than non-alcoholics (CI = 1.50 - 12.99; p = 0.017). (See table XV)

In the study conducted by Inge K. Hong et al, subjects with a history of alcoholism were 2.90 times more likely to die than non-alcoholics (CI :1.67 - 5.04) . (37)

4.2.5. Notion of asthma

In our study, univariate analysis showed that asthmatics were 7.83 times more likely to die during the intensive phase of treatment than non-asthmatics. However, multivariate analysis did not show this relationship. (See table XV)

In the study conducted by H. Gharsalli et al in Tunisia in 2014, 4 out of 10 patients who had both asthma and tuverculosis developed an asthma exacerbation during the course of the anti-tuberculosis treatment prescribed for all patients . (38)

The association between asthma and tuberculosis poses therapeutic problems due to interactions between anti-tuberculosis drugs and asthma drugs. (38; 39)

4.2.6. HIV serology

Our study showed that people living with HIV (PLHIV) were 3.62 times more likely to die (CI = 1.21 - 11.85; p = 0.004) (See Table XV).

Osman Abdullahi et al, in Kenya in 2017, found that HIV is a risk factor for mortality during TB treatment. In their study PLHIV on ART had 3.06 times the risk of dying than HIV-negative subjects (CI: 2.38-3.94) and PLHIV not on ART had a relative risk of 6.12 (CI: 3.15-11.89). (6) . Peter Seah Keng Tok et al, demonstrated a statistically significant relationship between HIV infection and mortality during tuberculosis treatment. In their study, PLHIV were more likely to die than HIV-negative subjects .(31)

HIV infection is the most important known risk factor for active TB in patients with TB infection. This risk is reduced when the HIV-infected person is on effective antiretroviral therapy (ART) (26) . Human immunodeficiency virus (HIV) infection and TB, which accelerate each other's progression, form a lethal association(3) . For some, the excess mortality among HIV-positive TB sufferers is due to the progression of the infection itself, to drug intolerance or treatment discontinuation, and to the fact that two serious diseases are progressing in the same person .(40; 41)

4.2.7. Consultation period

In our series, subjects with a consultation delay $\leq$ 30 days reduced the risk of dying in the intensive treatment phase of tuberculosis by 57% (CI = 0.22 - 0.88; $p = 0.036$). On the other hand, those with a consultation delay > 30 days multiplied this risk by 2.32. (See Table XV)

Hicham Janah et al, in Morocco in 2014, demonstrated in their study that a delay in diagnosis of more than 60 days is a risk factor for mortality in pulmonary tuberculosis . (19)

This is because these patients arrive at hospital with advanced disease.

4.2.8 Clinical manifestations

In our study, dyspnoea, haemoptysis, vertigo, pallor, bed rest and profound impairment of general condition were significantly associated with mortality during the intensive phase. Multivariate analysis did not show a relationship between haemoptysis and death during TB treatment. However, dyspnoea (RR = 1.92; CI = 1.84 - 6.41; $p = 0.012$), pallor (RR = 2.41; CI = 1.51 - 8.35; $p = 0.027$), vertigo (RR = 2.32; CI = 1.42 - 14.12; $p = 0.036$), bed rest (RR = 1.7; CI = 1.43 - 13.15 ; $p = 0.028$) and profound deterioration in general condition (RR = 3.01; CI = 1.42 - 6.38; p = 0.004) were shown to be risk factors for mortality during treatment of tuberculosis in the multivariate analysis. (See Table XV)

Harouna AML et al, in Senegal in 2019, found that dyspnoea was significantly associated with death (p = 0.001) (42) . Hicham Janah et al, working on risk factors for pulmonary tuberculosis mortality in Morocco in 2014, found that there was a statistically significant association between haemoptysis and death during tuberculosis treatment (19) . Haemoptysis may be one of the causes of anaemia, which could explain this risk of death.

Pallor and dizziness are clinical manifestations of anaemia. Anemia is a proven risk factor for mortality in several studies .(18; 37)

Dyspnoea is related to the age of the disease and the extent of damage to the lung parenchyma, which is not conducive to good haematosis(3) . Similarly, the profound deterioration in general condition is linked to the age and advanced stage of the disease.

4.3 Body mass index

Our study showed that patients with a BMI of less than 18.5 kg/m^2were 2.08 times more likely to die during the intensive phase of TB treatment (CI = 1.46 - 5.55; p = 0.039).

Osman Abdullahi et al, found that subjects with a BMI of less than 18.5 kg/m^2were 1.46 times more likely to die during tuberculosis treatment (CI: 1.39-1.53).

This could be explained by the fact that undernutrition is associated with malabsorption of the main anti-tuberculosis drugs .(43)

CONCLUSION AND RECOMMENDATIONS

1. Conclusion

Mortality during the intensive phase of tuberculosis is high, at 11.11%.

Age > 55, consultation > 30 days, smoking, alcoholism, dyspnoea, pallor, dizziness, bed rest, profound deterioration in general condition, positive HIV serology and BMI < 18.5 kg/m^{2}were the risk factors for mortality in the intensive phase of tuberculosis treatment. Patients with these characteristics need to be monitored with particular care, or even referred to a centre of excellence, to reduce the number of deaths.

2. Recommendations

We recommend the following:

3. Ministry of Health

1. Regularly provide the various TDCs with the equipment they need to screen for HIV, which is a major risk factor for mortality during the intensive phase of tuberculosis treatment;
2. Carry out large-scale studies to determine these factors in the provinces and in the country as a whole;
3. Raise awareness among the general public and carers of the risk factors for tuberculosis mortality so that these factors can be properly managed;
4. Draw up a mortality risk factor surveillance score and make it available to the various CDTs for surveillance of cases of tuberculosis and action to be taken in the case of tuberculosis patients presenting risk factors.

Nursing staff

1. Ensure close and rigorous monitoring of tuberculosis patients who present one of the risk factors for mortality, especially during the intensive phase of tuberculosis treatment;
2. Providing nutritional care for patients with a BMI < 18.5 kg/m^2;
3. Refer all patients with any risk factor for mortality to a specialist facility for holistic management.

Bibliography

1. WHO. *Global tuberculosis report 2021.* Geneva: s.n., 2021. ISBN 978-92-4-004162-2 (electronic version).

2. WHO. *Global tuberculosis report 2020: executive summary.* Geneva: s.n., 2020. ISBN 978-92-4-001696-5 (electronic version).

3. WHO. *Global tuberculosis control report 2018.* Geneva: s.n., 2018.

4. WHO. *World health statistics 2022: monitoring health for the SDGs, sustainable development goals.* 2022. ISBN 978-92-4-005114-0 (electronic version).

5. WHO. *WHO DRC.* [Online] 2022 March 24 [Citation : 08 07 2023] https://www.afro.who.int/fr/countries/democratic-republic-of-congo/news/la-rdc....

6. Osman A. Abdullahi, Moses M. Ngari, Deche Sanga, et al. *Mortality during treatment for tuberculosis; areview of surveillance data in a rural county in Kenya.* Kenya: PLOS ONE, July 11, 2019. https://doi.org/10.1371/journal.pone.0219191.

7. Adamu AL, Gadanya MA, Abubakar IS, Jibo AM, Bello MM, Gajida AU, et al. *High mortality amongtuberculosis patients on treatment in Nigeria: a retrospective cohort study. BMC infectious diseases.* s.l. : BMC infectious diseases, 2017; . https://doi.org/10.1186/s12879-017-2249-4 PMID: 28231851; PubMed Central PMCID: PMC5324260.

8. Takarinda KC, Sandy C, Masuka N, Hazangwe P, Choto RC, Mutasa-Apollo T, et al. *Factors Associated with Mortality among Patients on TB Treatment in the Southern Region of Zimbabwe.* s.l.. : Pubmed, 2017. .

https://doi.org/10.1155/2017/6232071 PMID: 28352474; PubMed Central PMCID: PMC5352882 publication of this paper..

9. Harries AD, Hargreaves NJ, Kemp J, Jindani A, Enarson DA, Maher D, et al. *Deaths from tuberculosis in sub-Saharan African countries with a high prevalence of HIV-1.* s.l.. Lancet, 2001. 357(9267):1519-23. https://doi.org/10.1016/S0140-6736(00)04639-0 PMID: 11377627.

10. Cazabon D, Alsdurf H, Satyanarayana S, Nathavitharana R, Subbaraman R, Daftary A, et al. *Quality of tuberculosis care in high burden countries: the urgent need to address gaps in the care cascade.* . s.l. : Int J Infect Dis, 2017. 56:111-6. https://doi.org/10.1016/j.ijid.2016.10.016 PMID: 27794468; PubMed Central PMCID: PMC5346036.

11. Hanson CL, Osberg M, Brown J, Durham G, Chin DP. *Conducting Patient-Pathway Analysis to Inform Programming of Tuberculosis Services: Methods.* s.l.. : J Infect Dis, 2017. :S679-S85. https://doi.org/10.1093/infdis/jix387 PMID: 29117350; PubMed Central PMCID: PMC5853893.

12. LOFOLI B. *Determinants of mortality in tuberculosis-HIV/AIDS coinfection in Kisangani.* s.l.. Memoire de fin d'étude inédit FMP; UNIKIS, 2018.

13. Shastri S, Naik B, Shet A, Rewari B, De Costa A. *TB treatment outcomes among TB-HIV co-infections in Karnataka, India: how do these compare with non-HIV tuberculosis outcomes in the province?* . s.l.. : BMC Public Health, 2013. 13 : 838..

14. Sileshi B, Deyessa N, Girma B, Melese M, Suarez P. *Predictors of mortality among TB-HIV co-infected patients being treated for tuberculosis*

in Northwest Ethiopia: a retrospective cohort study. s.l.. : BMC Infectious Diseases, 2013. 13 : 297..

15. Zachariah R, Spielmann MP, Harries AD, Salaniponi FML. *Moderate to severe malnutrition in patients with tuberculosis a risk factor associated with early death.* . s.l. : Trans Roy Soc Trop Med Hyg , 2002 . 96 : 291-4..

16. N. Lefebvre, and D.Falzon,. *Risk factors for death among tuberculosis cases: analysis of European surveillance data.* s.l. EUROPEAN RESPIRATORY JOURNAL, 2008. DOI: 10.1183/09031936.00131107.

17. I.S. Pradipta, N. van't Boveneind-Vrubleuskaya, et al. *Predictors for treatment outcomes among patients with drug-susceptible tuberculosis in the Netherlands: a retrospective cohort study.* Netherlands: Elsevier, 2018. https://doi.org/10.1016/j.cmi.2018.10.009.

18. Gelaw, et al. *Anemia as a risk factor for tuberculosis: a systematic review and meta-analysis.* Gondar, Ethiopia: Environmental Health and Preventive Medicine, 2021. https://doi.org/10.1186/s12199-020-00931-z.

19. Hicham Janah, Hicham Souhi, Hatim Kouismi, Karima Mark, et al,. *Risk factors for pulmonary tuberculosis mortality.* Rabat, Morocco: Pan African Medical Journal, 2014. ISSN: 1937- 8688, http://www.panafrican-med-journal.com/content/article/19/347/full/.

20. Adil Sbayi, Amine Arfaoui, Hasna Janah, Safaa EL Koraichi, et al. *Epidemiological characteristics and some risk factors.* Larache, Morocco : Pan African Medical Journal, of extrapulmonary tuberculosis in Larache, Morocco. ISSN: 1937-8688; 36(381). 10.11604/pamj.2020.36.381.24870; https://www.panafrican-med-journal.com//content/article/36/381/full.

21. Muhammad Osman, Cari van Schalkwyk, et al. *Mortality during tuberculosis treatment in South Africa using an 8-year analysis of the national tuberculosis treatment register.* s.l. Scientific Reports, 2021. | https://doi.org/10.1038/s41598-021-95331-w.

22. Henegar C., Behets F.,Vanden Driessche K., Tabala M. ,Bahati E.,Bola V.,Van Rie A. *Mortality among tuberculosis patients in the Democratic Republic of Congo.* s.l. : INT J TUBERC LUNG DIS , 2012. http://dx.doi.org/10.5588/ijtld.11.0613 16(9):1199-1204.

23. LILOLO Olivine. *Determinants of tuberculosis mortality in the city of Kisangani.* Kisangani: UNIKIS diploma thesis, 2018.

24. PNLT RDC. *Guide de prise en charge de la tuberculose PATI V.* s.l. Ministry of Health, National Tuberculosis Control Programme (PNLT), 2015.

25. MBO, JP. *Note de cours de Pneumologie.* Kisangani: Cours Inédit D1 Médecine FMP UNIKIS, 2019.

26. PNLT RDC. *Guide de prise en charge de la tuberculose PATI VI.* s.l. Ministry of Health, National Tuberculosis Control Programme (PNLT), 2020.

27. Waitt CJ, Peter K, Banda N, White SA, Kampmann B, Kumwenda J, Heyderman RS, Pirmohamed M, Squire SB. *Early deaths during tuberculosis treatment are associated with depressed innate responses, bacterial infection, and tuberculosis progression.* . s.l. : J Infect Dis, 2011. 204(3):358-62.

28. Bisson GP, Zetola N, Collman RG. *Persistent high mortality in advanced HIV/TB despite appropriate antiretroviral and antitubercular therapy: an emerging challenge.*. s.l.. : Current HIV/AIDS Reports, 2015. 12(1):107-16.

29. Pepper DJ, Rebe K, Morroni C, Wilkinson RJ, Meintjes G. *Clinical deterioration during antitubercular treatment at a District Hospital in South Africa: the importance of drug resistance and AIDS defining illnesses.* s.l. PLoS One, 2009. 4(2):e4520..

30. Gupta A, Nadkarni G, Yang WT, Chandrasekhar A, Gupte N, Bisson GP, Hosseinipour M, Gummadi N. *Early mortality in adults initiating antiretroviral therapy (ART) in low- and middle-income countries (LMIC): a systematic review and meta-analysis.* s.l. : PLoS One, 2011. 6:e28691.

31. Peter Seah Keng Tok, Su May Liew, Li Ping Wong, et al. *Determinants of unsuccessful treatment outcomes and mortality among tuberculosis patients in Malaysia: A registry-based cohort study.* Malaysia : PLOS ONE, April 22, 2020. https://doi.org/10.1371/journal.pone.0231986.

32. Poverty by qualification. [Online] 18 April 2023. [Citation : 29 06 2023.] https://www.inegalites.fr/La-pauvrete-selon-le-diplome#:~:text=Selon%20les%20donn%C3%A9es%202019%20de,(4%2C6%20%25)..

33. Moummi, Ahmed. *Analysis of Poverty in the Republic.* Tunis, Tunisia: Working Papers Series No. 112, African Development Bank (AfDB), 2010.

34. K. Adjoh, G. Ouedraogo S. Adambounou, A.R. Ouedraogo et al,. *Factors associated with deaths in tuberculosis patients in the intensive phase of treatment at the Sylvanus Olympio University Hospital in Lomé.* Lomé: Elsevier Masson, 2016. http://dx.doi.org/10.1016/j.rmr.2016.10.554.

35. Antoine D, Che D. *Tuberculosis cases reported in France in 2007.* s.l. Les cas de tuberculose déclarés en France, 2005. Available at https://www.ncbi.nlm.nih.gov/entrez/query.fcgi?db=PubMed&cmd=Search&doptcmdl=Citation&defaultField=Title+Word&term=Antoine%20D%5bauthor%5d+AND++Les+cas+de+tuberculose+dclars+en+France+en+2005.

36. Bulckaen H, Delaere S, Audubert E, Bout JC, Puisieux F, Dewailly P. *Factteurs pronostiques de la tuberculose du sujet âgé.* s.l. : Rev Med Interne. 2002, 2002. Available at: https://www.ncbi.nlm.nih.gov/entrez/query.fcgi?db=PubMed&cmd=Search&doptcmdl=Citation&defaultField=Title+Word&term=Bulckaen%20H%5bauthor%5d+AND++Prognostic+factors+for+tuberculosis+in+the+elderly+subject+g.

37. Inge K. Holden, Troels Lillebaek, Niels Seersholm5, Peter H. Andersen, et al. *Predictors for Pulmonary Tuberculosis Treatment Outcome in Denmark 2009-2014.* Denmark: Scientific Reports, 2019. (2019) 9:12995 | https://doi.org/10.1038/s41598-019-49439-9.

38. H. Gharsalli, S. Mokkadem, S. Aouadi , O. Neffati , A. Bayoudh , E. Mnif , M. Attia , S. Maalej , L. Douik Elgharbi. *Interaction between asthma and tuberculosis: about 10 cases.* Tunis : Journal of respiratory diseases, 2014. Doi : 10.1016/j.rmr.2014.10.456 .

39. L. Fekih, L. Boussoffara, M. Jemaa, S. Fenniche, H. Hassene, D. Belhabib, M.L. Megdiche. *Asthma and tuberculosis: beneficial association or evil?* . Tunis : Revue des maladies respiratoires, 2010. Doi : 10.1016/j.rmr.2010.06.010 .

40 KAZADI, Daniel. *Epidemiological, diagnostic, therapeutic and evolutionary aspects of tuberculosis-HIV/AIDS coinfection.* Kisangani: Memoire de Spécialisation FMP Kisangani, 2016.

41. Cox H., Hughes J., Daniels J., Azevedo V., et al. *Community-based treatment of drug-resistant tuberculosis in Khayelitsha, South Africa.* . s.l. : Int J Tuberc Lung Dis, 2014. 18:4418..

42. Harouna AML, Doutchi M, Amadou O, Abdou Neino M, Kadri S, Garba, Ndour CT. *Factteurs Prédictifs de Décès au Cours de la TuberculosePulmonaire chez les Patients Vivant avec le VIH au CNHU Fann de Dakar.* s.l. : Health Sci. Dis: Vol 20 , February 2019 . Available at www.hsd-fmsb.org.

43. WHO. *Guideline: Nutritional care and support for patients with Tuberculosis,.* Geneva : s.n., 2013.

Table of contents

INTRODUCTION 6
Chapter I: General information on tuberculosis 11
Chapter II: MATERIALS AND METHODS 28
Chapter III: RESULTS 33
Chapter IV: DISCUSSION 53
CONCLUSION AND RECOMMENDATIONS 60

APPENDIX

DATA COLLECTION FORM

CSDT name: ....

ADMISSION PROCEDURE: Consulted at the CDT

or Referral

by : ....

I. PATIENT IDENTITY

Name and Post-name
Age: Sex: Marital status :
Occupation: Employer :
Level of education: Religion :
Address :...
Tel:

II. HISTORY OF CURRENT ILLNESS

Start date of the first TBC events: ....
Circuit (Specify order of structures): ....
....
Health facilities consulted:...
Other structures consulted: Church
Traditional practitioner
Other
Date of first consultation at the CDT: ....
Number of days between onset of illness and first visit to CDT :

III. BACKGROUND

Notion of contagion: Yes
No
Relationship :
Notion of smoking: Yes
No
Duration :
Quantity :
Notion of smoking: Yes
No
Duration :
Quantity :
Diabetes
Drop
Asthma
HIV
Heart disease
Other (please specify):..

IV. CLINICAL MANIFESTATIONS

Symptoms on admission

SIGNS	Yes	No	Duration (months/days)	OBSERVATION
Respiratory signs				
Cough				
Sputum				
Dyspnoea				
Chest pain				
General signs				
Fever				
Physical asthenia				
Anorexia				
Weight loss				
Night sweats				
Pallor				
Vertigo				
Diarrhoea				
Bedridden				
Ambulante				

Other (please specify):...

...

RADIOLOGICAL SIGNS

Nature and extent of injuries				
a) Nature				
Opacity				
Infiltrates				
Opacity + infiltrates				
Nodules				
Military				
Cavern				
Tuberculous lobitis				
Other				
b) Scope				
Minime				
Large				

Other radiological signs to be specified:...

...

PHYSICAL SIGNS EN: cpm

SIGNS	Yes	No	OBSERVATION
Profound alteration of the EG			
Ascites			
Adenopathy			Cervical Axillary Inguinale General Other: ....
Hepatomegaly			
Splenomegaly			
Jaundice			

Other (please specify):...

....

V. FORM OF TUBERCULOSIS

Pulmonary : BK+ BK -
TOE : BK+ BK -
Type of PET: Military
Pericarditis
Pleuresis
Pot sickness
White tumour
Coxalgia
Ganglion
Other to be specified :

VI. PARACLINIQUES

Spitting :

- Zhiel : Positive Negative Number of crosses
- Auramine : Positive Negative Number of crosses
- Genexpert :Positive Negative Number of crosses

Blood glucose: Blood count: Hb :
HIV serology: HIV positive HIV negative Indeterminate :
If PHA (CD4 count) :
Other examinations to be specified:..

VII. ANTI-TUBERCULOSIS AND OTHER TREATMENTS

CATEGORY OF TREATMENT: New case :

Case already dealt with:

Date of start of anti-tuberculosis treatment
If HIV positive: NC screened at CDT
Already on ARVs
Date of start of ARV treatment:...../....../............
Number of days after starting ARV treatment :
Other treatment:

COMPLIANCE WITH TREATMENT

DOT : Yes
No
Type of DOT: CDT :
Community
If HIV positive: ARV :
Yes
No
Other medicines :

FOLLOW-UP CARE: Inpatient care

Ambulatory

EVOLUTION UNDER TREATMENT

Usual weight: Kg Weight at first consultation: kg Height: BMI :

Month	M1	M2	M3
Weight	kg	kg	kg

Side-effects: Yes No Occurred on .... day of treatment.

Describe :

Duration of disappearance of fever :

OUTCOME OF TREATMENT

Survivor

Deaths

Abandon

Transferred

TIME OF DEATH

- Date of death :
- Time interval between start of anti-tuberculosis treatment and death :
- Time interval between the start of ART and death :
- Cause of death :

FSC
www.fsc.org
MIX
Papier | Fördert gute Waldnutzung
FSC® C083411

Kolibri 360 GmbH
Ferdinand-Jühlke-Straße 7
99095 Erfurt, Deutschland
produktsicherheit@kolibri360.de

Druck:
CPI Druckdienstleistungen GmbH
im Auftrag der
Kolibri 360 GmbH
Ferdinand-Jühlke-Str. 7
99095 Erfurt